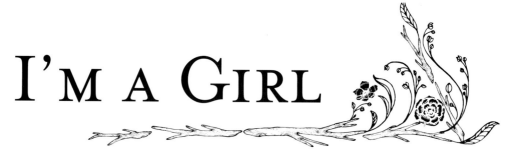

I'M A GIRL

MY CHANGING BODY!

Describes the early signs of puberty

BY
SHELLEY METTEN, M.S., PH.D.
WITH ALAN ESTRIDGE

ILLUSTRATION BY
KAREN WANG & JESSIE DO

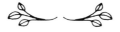

"OUR GOAL IS THAT CHILDREN EVERYWHERE WILL HAVE THE KNOWLEDGE
TO MAKE WISE CHOICES IN THE CARE OF THEIR BODIES."
-DR. METTEN, ANATOMY FOR KIDS®

For Brooke, my daughter-in-law,
a caring and compassionate woman
who has stolen my heart.

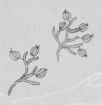

ISBN -13:978-0-9895469-8-0
SECOND EDITION

VISIT US AT WWW.ANATOMYFORKIDS.COM

REPRODUCTIVE SYSTEM SERIES FOR GIRLS

The I'm a Girl Series consists of five books and provides young girls with the knowledge they need to understand the maturing features of their reproductive system. It helps answer the question "why" the changes are happening.

I'M A GIRL: SPECIAL ME *(Ages 5-7)*

This book is intended to prepare young girls as they enter puberty in just a few years. It introduces the concept of where babies come from. This book will be of particular interest to a young girl whose mother is pregnant or has recently given birth. It also emphasizes the importance for young girls to protect themselves from inappropriate touching.

I'M A GIRL: MY CHANGING BODY *(Ages 8-9)*

There are two books that describe the changes a young girl experiences during puberty. This book is intended for a young girl in early puberty who has begun to notice changes in her breasts, a change in body odor, and a change in her emotions.

I'M A GIRL: HORMONES! *(Ages 10+)*

This book about puberty prepares a young girl for her first menstrual period. It describes the fascinating time of hormones that usher in the menstrual cycle and the daily changes her body will experience.

I'M A GIRL: HOW ARE BOYS DIFFERENT? *(Ages 13+)*

This book is intended for girls who have learned about the changes in their own body as a result of puberty and want to compare it to the changes happening in a boy's body at a similar age.

I'M A GIRL: SEXUAL MATURITY *(Ages 15+)*

This book is intended for girls who have already begun their menstrual periods and have questions about reproduction. The content addresses conception, contraception, and reproductive health.

ALONG WITH A MULTIPLE BOOK SERIES, THE ANATOMY FOR KIDS® WEBSITE, FACEBOOK PAGE, AND YOUTUBE CHANNEL PROVIDE USEFUL RESOURCES TO SUPPORT PARENTS. THESE LEARNING RESOURCES ARE NOT INTENDED TO PROMOTE ANY SPECIFIC MORAL OR CULTURAL PERSPECTIVE. ANATOMY FOR KIDS® CONSIDERS THAT A PARENT OR OTHER CONCERNED ADULT WOULD PREFER TO PROVIDE THAT GUIDANCE THEMSELVES.

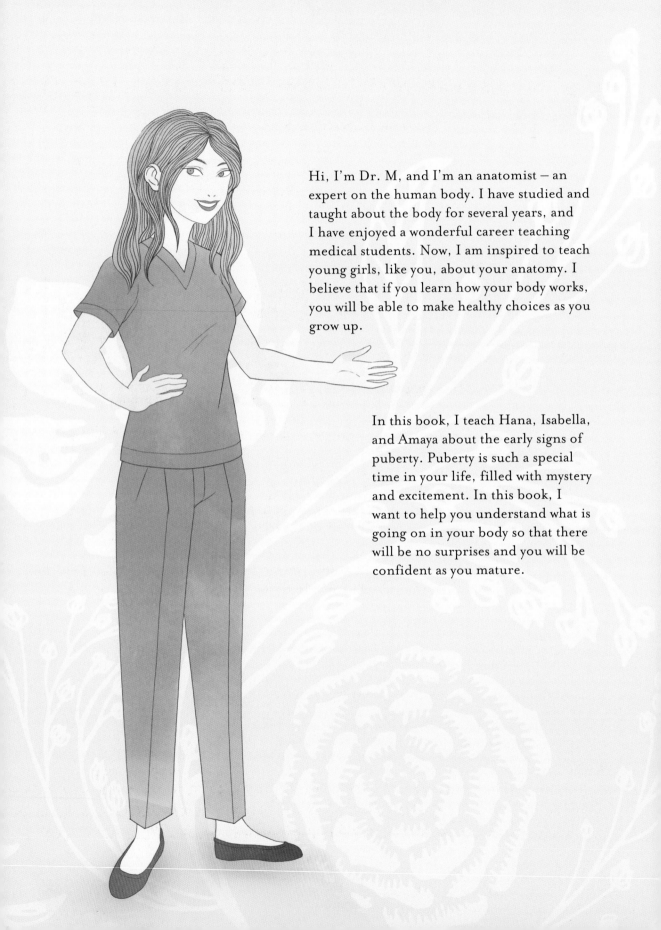

Hi, I'm Dr. M, and I'm an anatomist — an expert on the human body. I have studied and taught about the body for several years, and I have enjoyed a wonderful career teaching medical students. Now, I am inspired to teach young girls, like you, about your anatomy. I believe that if you learn how your body works, you will be able to make healthy choices as you grow up.

In this book, I teach Hana, Isabella, and Amaya about the early signs of puberty. Puberty is such a special time in your life, filled with mystery and excitement. In this book, I want to help you understand what is going on in your body so that there will be no surprises and you will be confident as you mature.

LOOKING FOR ANSWERS?

Words in **bold** in the text are defined under **Special Words** on pages 42-43.

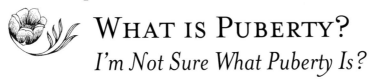 WHAT IS PUBERTY?
I'm Not Sure What Puberty Is?

"I did it!" shouted Isabella, showing Amaya her video game screen.

"You beat my high score!" said Amaya. They had been playing and talking for hours.

"Hey, Hana was telling me about **puberty** *(PEW-bur-tee)* the other day," said Amaya. "Have you heard of that?"

"No, what's puberty?" asked Isabella.

"It's something about our bodies. I think it has to do with what Dr. M taught us last year," replied Amaya.

"You mean about the eggs in the **ovaries** *(OH-vuh-rees)*?" asked Isabella.

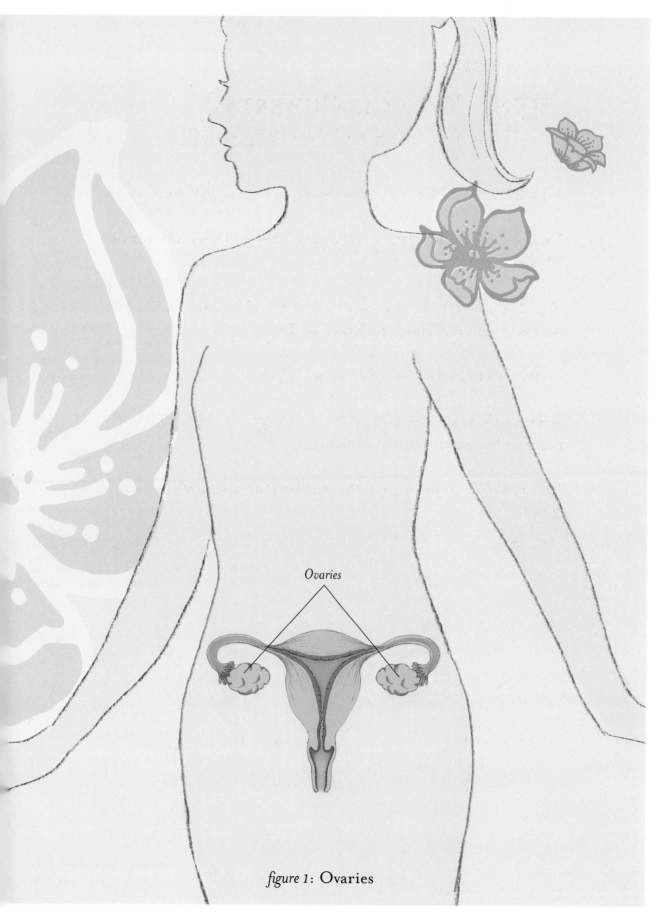

figure 1: Ovaries

9

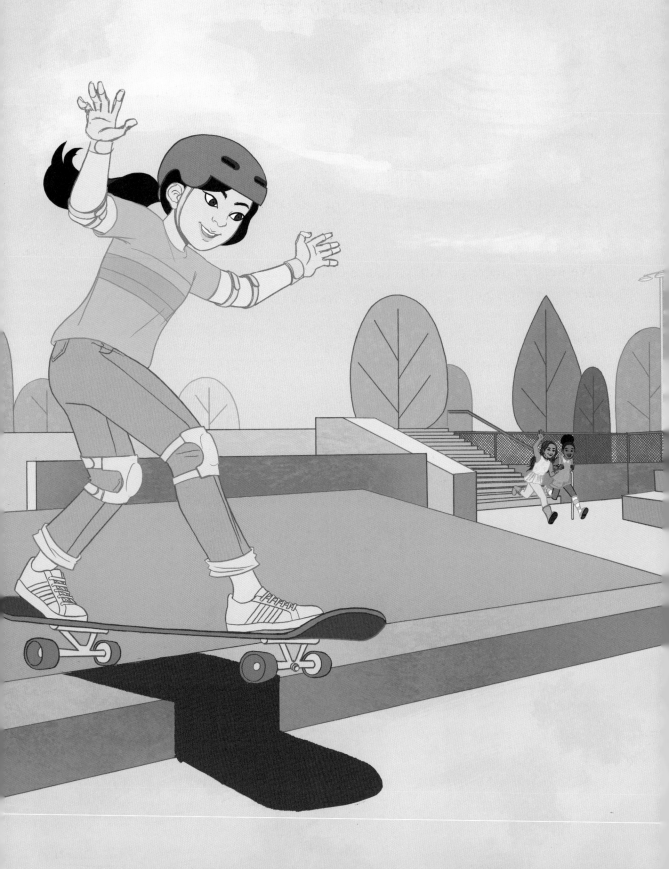

Is My Body Going to Start Changing Soon?

"Yeah," responded Amaya, "She also said there would be other changes. Hana thinks our bodies are going to start changing pretty soon."

"Whoa," said Isabella. "Maybe we should talk to Dr. M right away. We could ask her to teach us about puberty and what might happen to us next."

"We need Hana to go with us to see Dr. M," said Amaya. "She's at the skate park with her brother. Let's go find her."

The girls found Hana at the skate park and watched her in the half-pipe for a little while.

Isabella waved to Hana. "Nice run, Hana!"

"Thanks, Isabella. Whew! I'm pretty tired. I think I'm done for the day," said Hana, taking off her helmet.

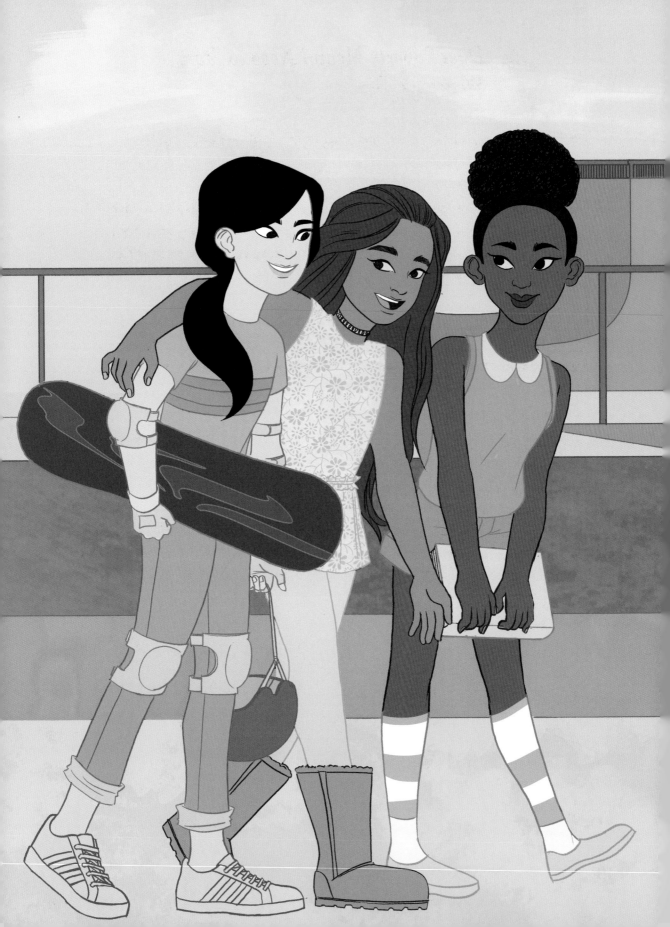

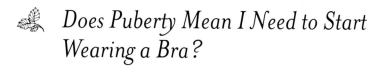 *Does Puberty Mean I Need to Start Wearing a Bra?*

"So I was telling Isabella what you told me the other day about puberty," said Amaya.

"Well, I don't know that much," said Hana. "I know it has to do with changes in our bodies, but I don't really know what that means. My friend Lakshmi started wearing a bra, and she said her mom told her it was because of puberty."

"We thought Dr. M could teach us about it," said Isabella.

"Great idea!" exclaimed Hana. "Let's ask our moms if we can go see her."

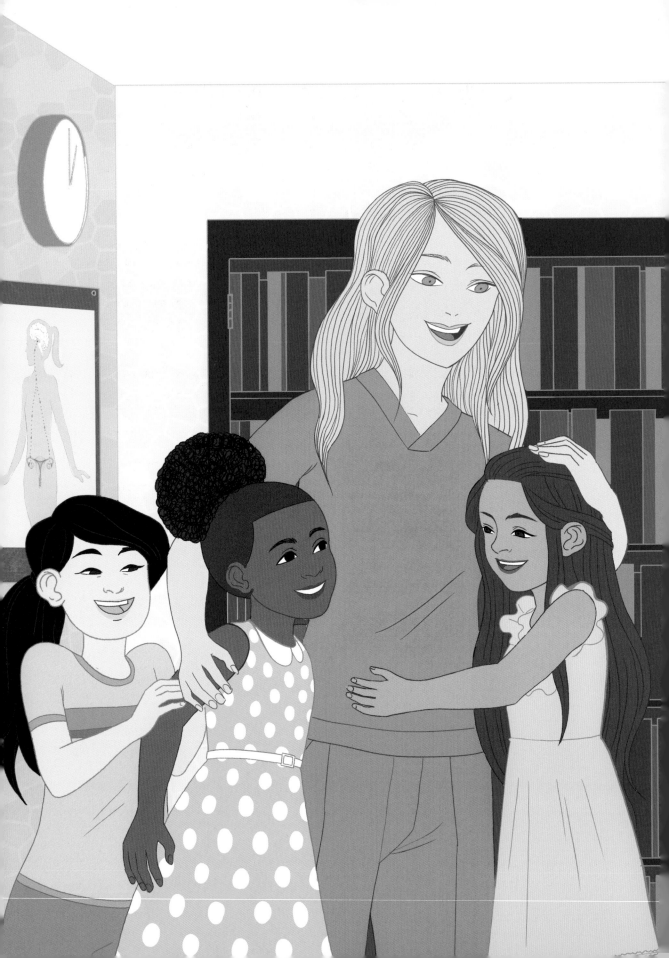

Why Do I Need to Go Through Puberty?

The next day the girls went to Dr. M's office. "Hi girls," greeted Dr. M. "It's so nice to see you again."

"Hi, Dr. M," said an enthusiastic Isabella. "We have lots of questions for you."

"We want to learn about puberty." exclaimed Amaya. "We think the changes you said were coming are starting to happen to us now. We've heard a lot of different things but we don't know anything about it."

"The best way to describe puberty is a time when your reproductive structures mature so that when you are older, you will be able to have a baby," explained Dr. M.

For most girls, puberty begins about 8 or 9 years old. It starts very quietly and you might not notice anything different in the beginning. Puberty lasts for a few years and during that time, there will be many changes in your body. But today we can talk about the early signs of puberty that you might be starting to notice or can expect in the near future.

Dr. M Says:

"Puberty prepares your body to be able to have a baby one day."

Chapter 2

OUTSIDE CHANGES
Why Do I Smell Different and Have Pimples on My Face?

"One of the first signs you might notice that puberty has begun is a change in your body odor," said Dr. M.

"I knew something was different when my mom took me to the store to buy deodorant!" said Hana.

Dr. M laughed. "Let me tell you something interesting about body odor. Everywhere in your skin are **sweat glands**. You have already noticed how sweaty you can get after skateboarding for a while."

What you might not know is there are bacteria that live on your skin, and it is okay for them to be there. In certain places in your body, like your armpits and around your private parts, are sweat glands that produce a special sweat that the bacteria like. They take in the sweat and produce a smelly gas that is your body odor.

Something else you might notice just as puberty starts is a change in the skin on your face. Little red bumps called **pimples** might begin to show up. It's a good idea to keep your face clean and not touch the pimples. They'll come and go over the next few years, but touching them can make the situation worse.

Dr. M Says:

"Two of the early signs of puberty are a change in your body odor and the appearance of pimples on your face."

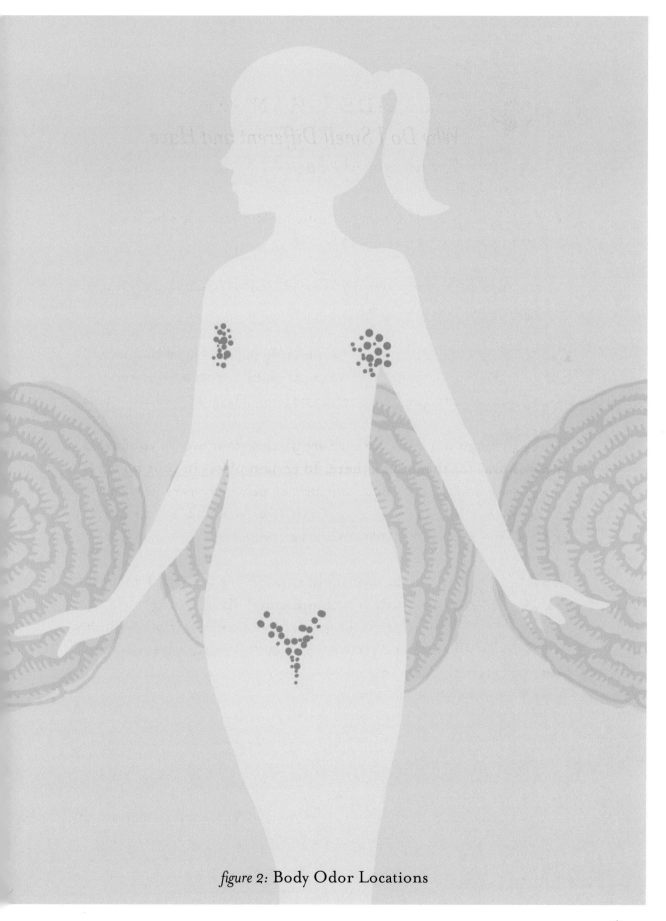

figure 2: Body Odor Locations

🌸 *Why are There Little Lumps in My Breasts?*

Soon, you will begin to feel some changes in your **breasts**. In this anatomy figure, notice the **nipple** is surrounded by a lighter colored circle called the **areola**. Each year the areola will become a little darker.

An early sign that puberty has started is when little lumps begin to form under your nipples. These little lumps are called **breast buds**.

"I think I already have breast buds," said Amaya, shyly. "I am so happy to know they are normal lumps in my breasts."

Breast buds are small balls of fat that surround tiny growing breast glands. They don't always grow in both breasts at the same time. You might find a few little lumps in one breast and then some weeks later, find them in the other breast too. This is normal.

While breast buds are growing, your nipples might feel tender. This is a good time to start wearing a soft cotton bra to decrease discomfort for your maturing nipples.

In the next few years, more fat will collect in your breasts and change the shape of your breasts until they are the shape seen in a teenager.

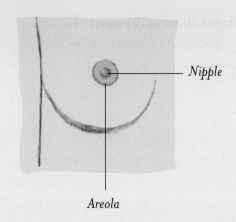

Nipple

Areola

figure 3a: Breast

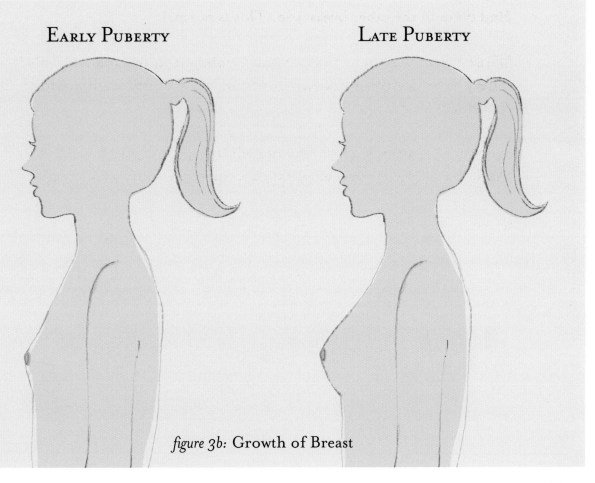

EARLY PUBERTY

LATE PUBERTY

figure 3b: Growth of Breast

Why Am I Growing Taller So Fast?

In the same way that fat begins to collect in your breasts and give them a different shape, fat also collects in other parts of your body during the early years of puberty.

You will likely notice that your face seems a little fuller and your clothes are tighter around the middle. Don't be concerned. If you are eating a good diet and exercising, you will soon grow taller and the shape of your body will change.

"I'm glad to hear that my body is just going through a stage, but I don't understand how my body grows taller," said Isabella.

Dr. M explained. "Your bones have patches in them called **growth plates** that you can see in this anatomy figure. As the growth plates grow, so do the bones. Look for the blue growth plates in the legs. As these growth plates grow more bone, the leg bones become longer and you become taller."

Dr. M Says:

"Breast buds under your nipples are normal changes in early puberty. Growth plates in your legs are the reason you grow taller."

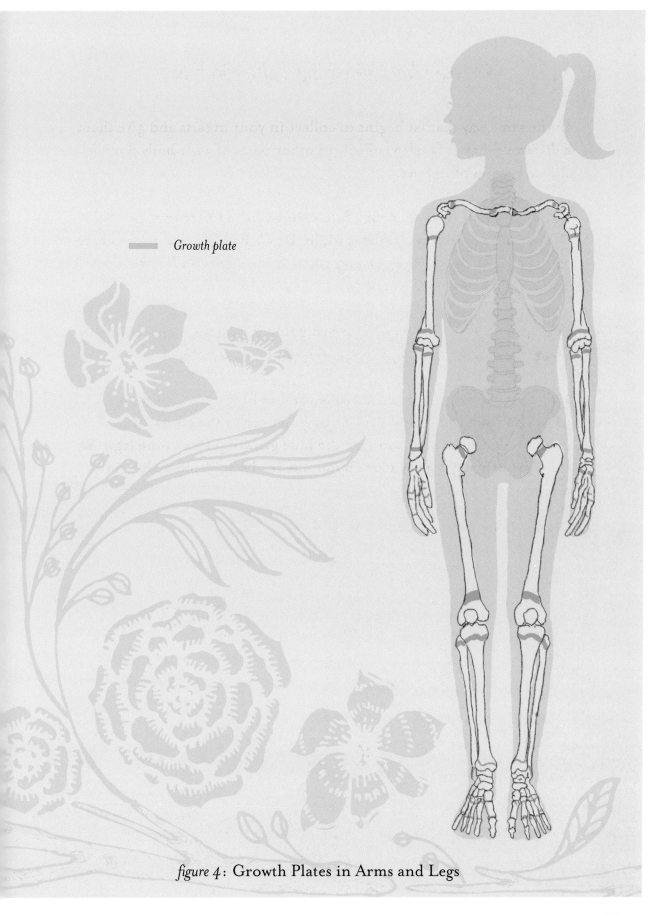

Growth plate

figure 4: Growth Plates in Arms and Legs

Chapter 3

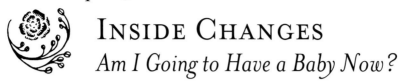 ## INSIDE CHANGES
Am I Going to Have a Baby Now?

"I understand that we go through puberty so we can have a baby one day, but I don't understand what is going to change inside of me," said Hana.

"I don't want to have a baby right now!" exclaimed a very concerned Amaya.

"Don't worry, Amaya," comforted Dr. M. "Your reproductive structures are still immature."

So that you can understand what changes are going to happen in your reproductive structures, let's learn about where these structures are located in your body and what they do.

If you put your hands on your hips, the bone you are touching is called the **pelvis**. The pelvis is a circle of bone with a big space in the middle called the **pelvic cavity**. There are reproductive structures tucked inside the pelvic cavity.

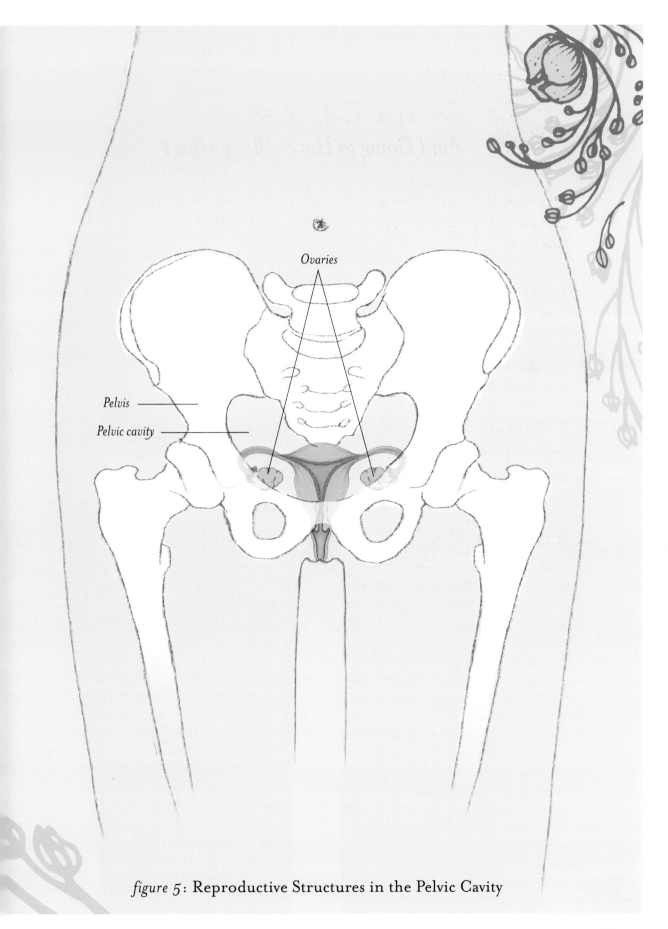

Ovaries

Pelvis

Pelvic cavity

figure 5: Reproductive Structures in the Pelvic Cavity

How Many Eggs Are in My Ovaries?

The pelvis has been hidden in this anatomy figure. Look for two **ovaries**. Ovaries are filled with **eggs**. There are about 300,000 eggs in your ovaries right now.

"Wow, that's a lot of eggs," exclaimed Isabella.

Later in puberty, your ovaries start to let go of their eggs, usually one at a time. It is called **ovulation** *(ah-view-LAY-shun)* when an egg leaves an ovary.

"What happens to the egg after it leaves my ovary?" asked Hana.

"Do you see the large triangular-shaped structure in the middle of the pelvic cavity? This is the **uterus** *(YOU-tur-us)*," explained Dr. M. "The egg is heading to the uterus."

Coming out of each side of the uterus is a long tube called a **fallopian** *(fuh-LOW-pee-an)* **tube**. On the end of the fallopian tube, near the ovary, are tiny finger-like structures that beat and direct the egg into the fallopian tube. The fallopian tube is the pathway for the egg to the uterus.

Dr. M Says:

"At ovulation, an egg leaves an ovary and enters the fallopian tube on its way to the uterus."

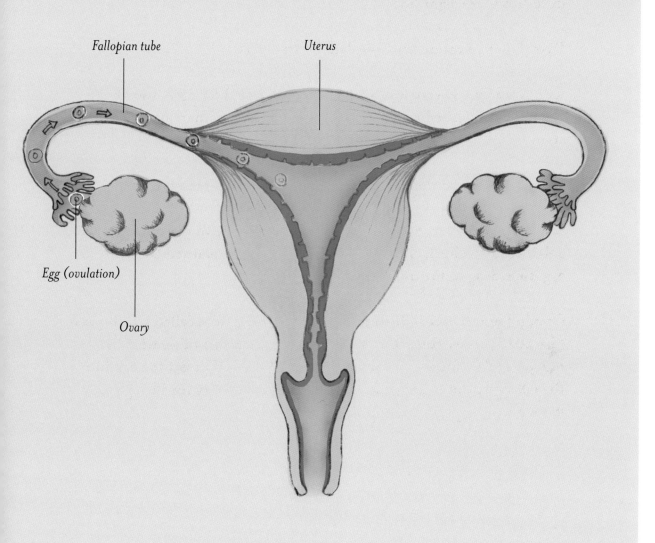

Fallopian tube

Uterus

Egg (ovulation)

Ovary

figure 6: Ovulation

🌸 What Happens to an Egg in the Uterus?

In this anatomy figure, you can see an **egg** leaving the **ovary** at **ovulation** and taking a four-day journey inside a **fallopian tube** to the **uterus**.

Notice that the uterus has a space in the middle called the **uterine** (*YOU-tur-in*) **cavity**. When the egg reaches the uterus, it goes into the uterine cavity. You don't see it anymore because it fades away and is gone.

Each month is just a practice run. These eggs cannot grow into a baby. Later, when an egg meets a sperm in the fallopian tube, the egg will grow into a baby inside the uterus.

Dr. M Says:
⁂

"After four days in the fallopian tube, the egg arrives in the uterine cavity and fades away."

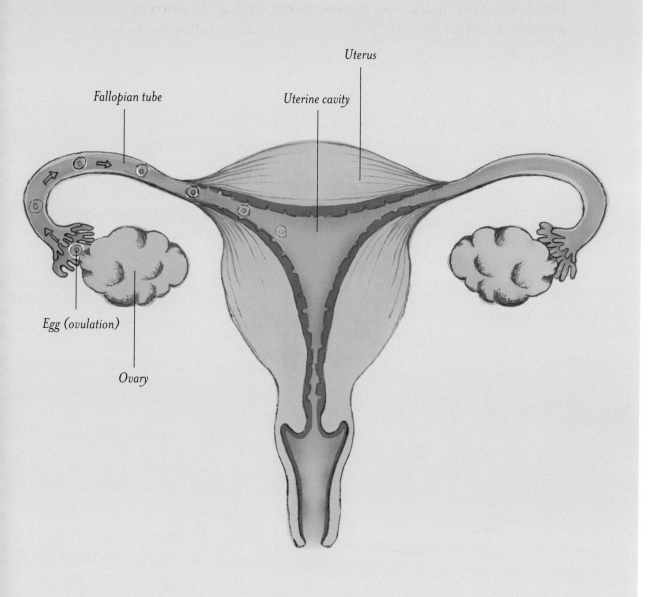

Uterus

Fallopian tube

Uterine cavity

Egg (ovulation)

Ovary

figure 7: Journey of the Egg

How Does a Baby Squeeze Through the Vagina to Get Out?

At one end of the **uterus** are the two **fallopian tubes**. At the other end of the uterus there is another tube called the **vagina** *(vuh-JINE-uh)*.

When a baby is being born, the thick walls of the uterus push the baby into the vagina. The vagina can stretch a lot so the baby has room to squeeze through and be born.

Notice there is an opening at the end of the vagina called the **vaginal** *(VA-juh-null)* **opening**. This is where the baby comes out.

Dr. M Says:

"The vagina is a tube that stretches to let a baby squeeze through. The baby pushes through the vaginal opening to be born."

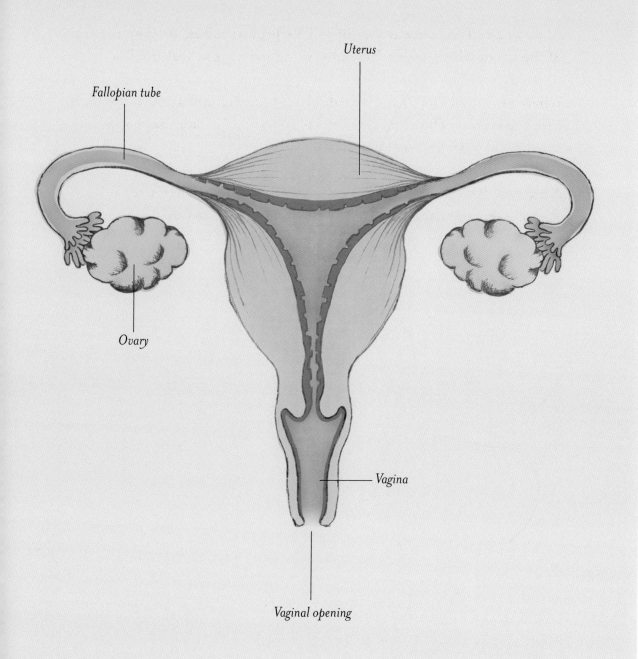

Fallopian tube

Uterus

Ovary

Vagina

Vaginal opening

figure 8: Vagina

❀ Where is the Uterus and Vagina in the Pelvic Cavity?

"This is a special anatomy figure that shows structures that are deep in the **pelvic cavity**," continued Dr. M. "It lets you peek inside the pelvic cavity from the side so you can see what structures live there."

"I see the **uterus**," observed Isabella. "Oh, and there is the **vagina** too."

"You can also see the **vaginal opening** where the baby comes out," explained Dr. M.

The uterus and vagina are in the middle of the pelvic cavity between two other structures that are not reproductive structures. They also live in the pelvic cavity.

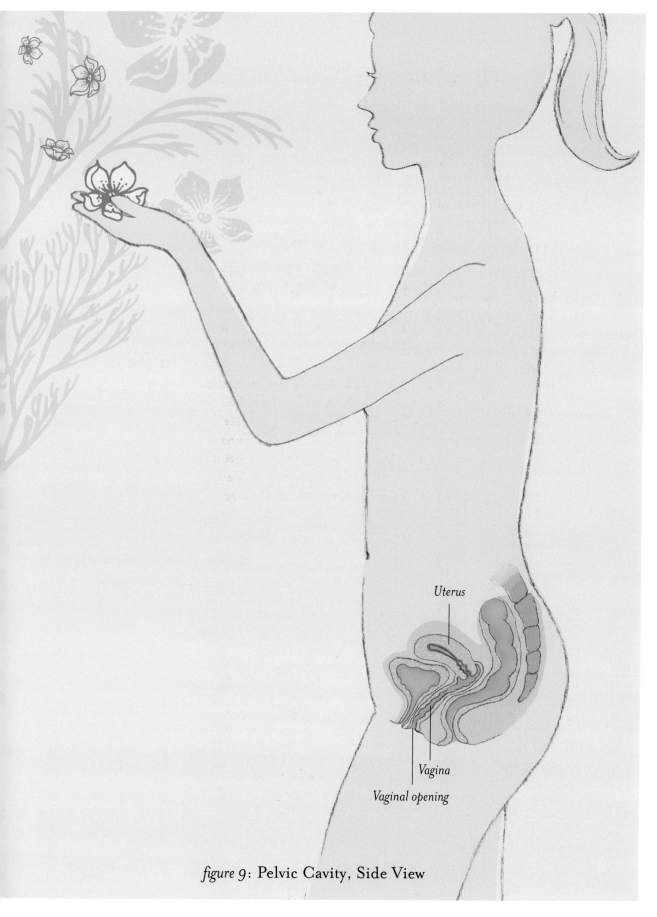

figure 9: Pelvic Cavity, Side View

🌹 *What Else is in The Pelvic Cavity?*

The **uterus** and **vagina** are in the middle. In front of them is the **urinary** *(UR-in-air-ee)* **bladder**. This is where urine is stored until you are ready to urinate, or pee.

Coming down from the urinary bladder is a little tube called the **urethra** *(you-REE-thruh)*. When you are ready to pee, the urinary bladder squeezes urine into the urethra.

The end of the urethra has an opening called the **urethral** *(you-REE-thrull)* **opening**. This is where pee comes out.

So there are two different openings:
- Pee comes out the urethral opening
- Babies come out the vaginal opening

"There is one more structure in the pelvic cavity that is not one of the reproductive structures," said Dr. M. "It is called the **rectum** and it is behind the uterus and vagina. It stores feces, or poop. The rectum squeezes the feces out an opening called the **anus**."

"Okay, that's way more than I wanted to know!" exclaimed Amaya.

Dr. M Says:
🙢🙠
"The uterus and vagina are in the middle of the pelvic cavity."

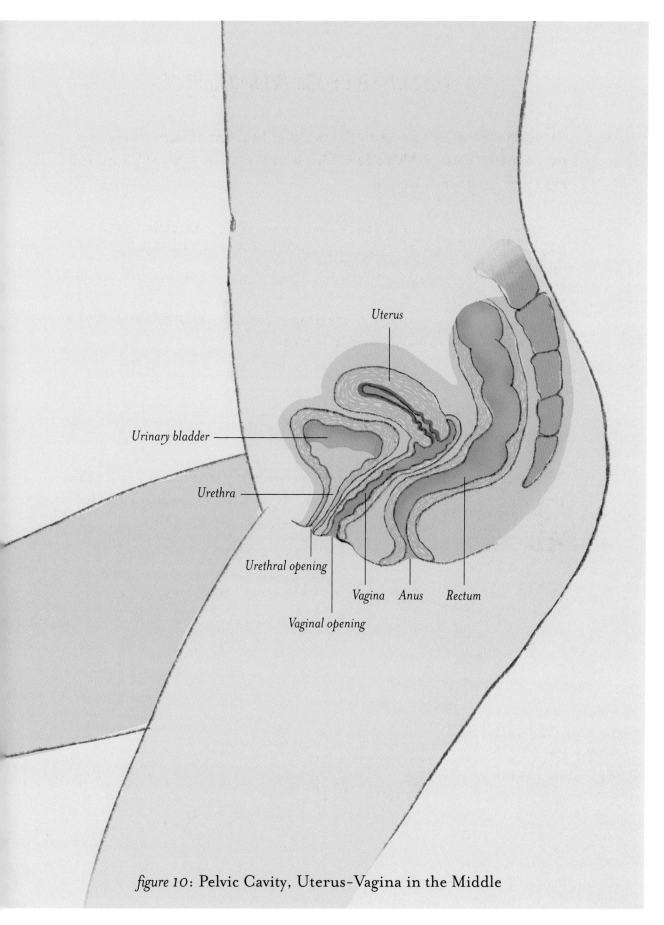

Uterus

Urinary bladder

Urethra

Urethral opening

Vaginal opening

Vagina   Anus   Rectum

figure 10: Pelvic Cavity, Uterus-Vagina in the Middle

Chapter 4

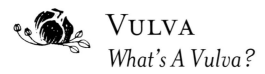

VULVA
What's A Vulva?

"A discussion about puberty would not be complete unless we talk about the **vulva** *(VUL-vuh)*," said Dr. M.

"What's a vulva?" asked Amaya suspiciously.

"The vulva," explained Dr. M, "is also called your private parts. It is located between your legs. The vulva is the part of your female anatomy that you can see."

Hana was feeling a little uncomfortable now. "I'm embarrassed talking about my private parts," she said.

Dr. M reassured the girls. "I know a lot of this is new to you. Talking about these things may feel a little strange at first, but it is important for you to know about all of your female anatomy, especially your private parts. The more you know, the less confused you will be about puberty."

And, it's always okay to talk to your parents or your doctor about these things. I am talking to you about this today because your parents asked if I would help explain all of this to you.

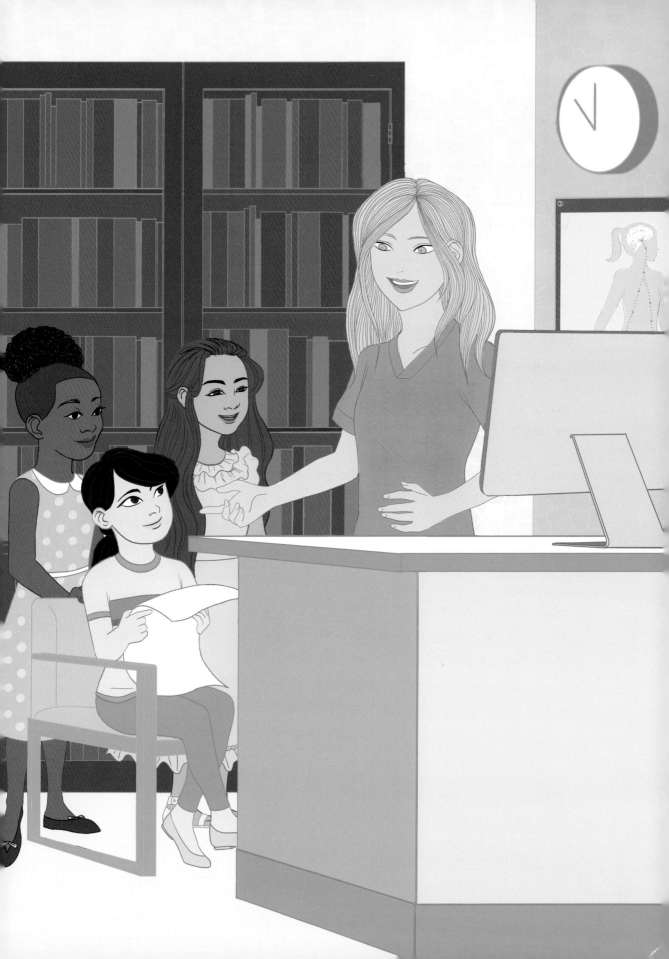

🌿 Do I Have Pubic Hair Now?

Another early sign of puberty that you might notice soon is tiny hairs growing on the outside of the **vulva**. These are called **pubic** *(PEW-bic)* **hair**. As you mature through puberty, your pubic hair will become curly, and there will be more and more hair.

Attached to pubic hair are the special sweat glands that make the fluid that bacteria like. The bacteria produce a body odor that you will notice near your vulva. It is important to keep the vulva clean.

"Dr. M," said Isabella. "I've been looking at this anatomy figure of the vulva, and I don't see where a baby would come out."

Hana groaned when Isabella said this. "Is there more?" she asked with caution.

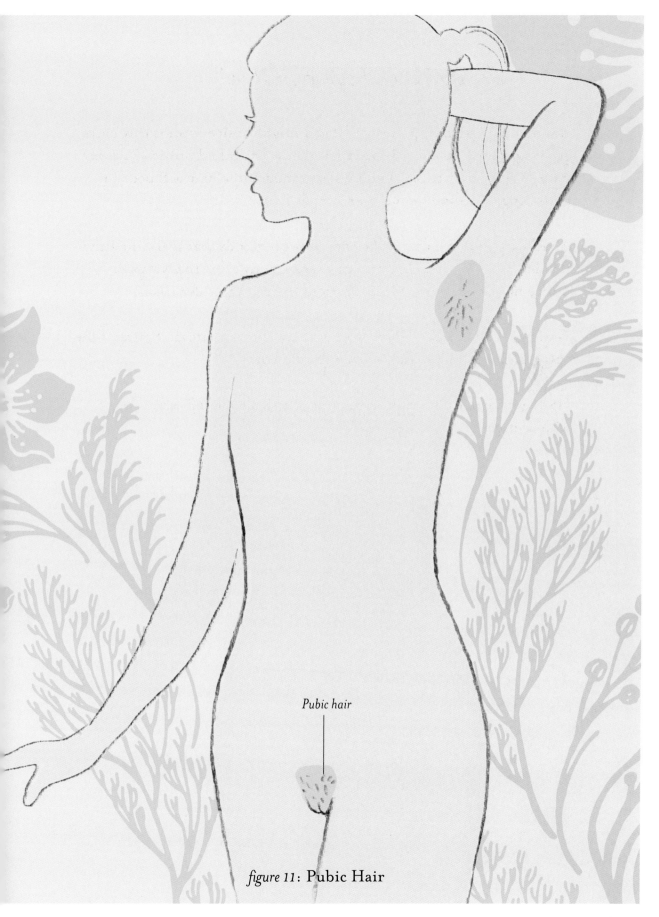

Pubic hair

figure 11: Pubic Hair

✎ Does a Baby and Pee Come Out the Same Opening in the Vulva?

"Yes, Hana," explained Dr. M. "There is more to learn about the vulva, but we need to look at a different anatomy figure."

"Okay, now I am very uncomfortable!" exclaimed Hana.

"The **vulva** is a very special part of our body and a part we don't often learn about," explained Dr. M. "It's okay to feel a little uncomfortable, but let's learn about what's there."

There are two openings you've already learned. The smaller opening above is called the **urethral opening**. This is where pee comes out. The larger opening below is the **vaginal opening**. This is where a baby comes out to be born.

"Okay, this is making more sense to me," said Isabella. "Now I see there is one opening for pee and one for the baby to come through."

Folding over these two openings to protect them are two thin folds of skin called the **labia** *(LAY-be-uh)* **minora** *(my-NOR-uh)*. On the outside of the vulva are two larger folds of skin called the **labia** *(LAY-be-uh)* **majora** *(muh-JOR-uh)*. The hair that is found on the outside of the vulva is given a special name. It is called **pubic** *(PEW-bic)* **hair**.

Dr. M Says:

❧⚜☙

"The vulva has two openings, the urethral opening and the vaginal opening. There are also two folds of skin that protect the vulva called the labia minora and labia majora."

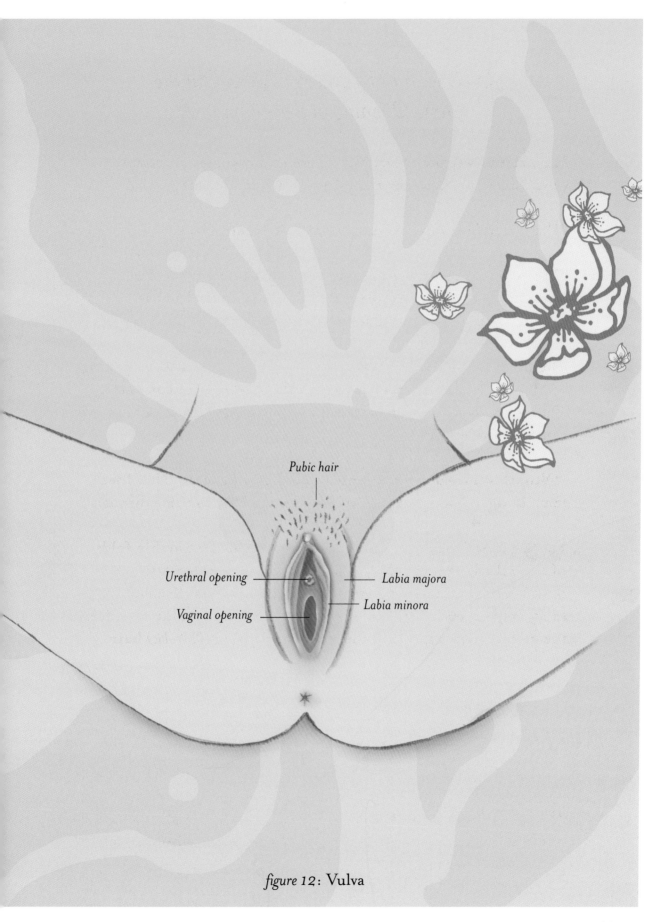

Pubic hair

Urethral opening ———○———— Labia majora

Vaginal opening ———————— Labia minora

figure 12: Vulva

Chapter 5

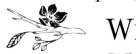 # WHAT'S NEXT
Why Do I Feel So Emotional?

"We have talked about several changes that happen in your body during the early days of puberty, but have you noticed a change in your emotions?" asked Dr. M.

"I know my brother is more irritating now, but I didn't think that was because of something changing about me," said Hana.

For the next few years, your brain is going to change a lot. The emotional part of your brain will be very powerful, while other parts that keep you calm are trying to catch up. One minute you might be laughing and happy, and then suddenly something happens and you are irritated or sad.

"I have a feeling there are more changes coming than what you told us about today," expressed Amaya.

"Yes, Amaya," responded Dr. M. "The changes we talked about today are ones you will notice in the next few months. There are other changes coming in the next few years."

When Is My Period Going To Start?

For example, **hormones** will make a big difference in your body and especially in your reproductive structures. Because of hormones, you will start having **menstrual** *(MEN-strull)* **periods**.

"I think I'm a little afraid of that happening to me," said Hana. "How will I know what to do? What if I'm at a skate park and I don't know if there is a bathroom there!"

We have some time before you start having your period. In a few months, let's plan another time for me to teach you about hormones and how to prepare for your first menstrual period.

"Thank you, Dr. M," expressed Isabella. "We are so happy to learn about the changes that are coming. Now, I feel like I'm prepared for anything."

"It is my pleasure and I look forward to seeing you again soon," replied Dr. M.

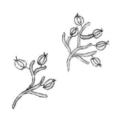

SPECIAL WORDS

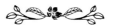

Breasts: nipple and **areola**

Breast buds: small mounds of fat that surround tiny breast glands under the nipple

Fallopian (*fuh-LOW-pee-an*) **tube:** there are two fallopian tubes; pathway for an egg from an ovary to the uterus. Finger-like processes on the ends guide an egg inside after ovulation.

Growth plates: small patches in the bone that grow and the bone becomes longer and bigger

Hormone: a chemical that travels in the blood and tells cells somewhere else in the body to perform different functions

Menstrual (*MEN-strull*) **period:** simply called your period. This is because of hormones.

Ovaries (*OH-vuh-rees*): two ovaries located in the pelvic cavity that contain about 300,000 **eggs** when puberty begins

Ovulation (*ah-view-LAY-shun*): when an egg leaves an ovary

Pelvis: a circle of bone that surrounds a space called the **pelvic cavity**. Important female reproductive structures are located in the pelvic cavity.

Pimple: small red bumps in the skin, mostly in the face

Puberty (*PEW-bur-tee*): prepares your female reproductive structures so you can have a baby one day

Pubic (*PEW-bic*) **hair:** hair that grows on parts of the vulva

Sweat glands: special clumps of cells in the skin that produce sweat

Urinary (*UR-in-air-ee*) **bladder:** stores urine and then sends it down the **urethra** (*you-REE-thruh*) and out the **urethral** (*you-REE-thrull*) **opening** in the vulva when you urinate

Uterus *(YOU-tur-us)*: reproductive structure in the pelvic cavity. There is a space in the center called the **uterine** *(YOU-tur-in)* **cavity**.

Vagina *(vuh-JINE-uh)*: reproductive structure in the pelvic cavity. It opens in the vulva as the **vaginal** *(VA-juh-null)* **opening**.

Vulva *(VUL-vuh)*: includes **urethral opening** and **vaginal opening**; also two skin flaps-**labia** *(LAY-be-uh)* **minora** *(my-NOR-uh)* and **labia** *(LAY-be-uh)* **majora** *(muh-JOR-uh)*

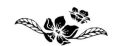

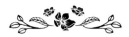

**AUTHOR
SHELLEY METTEN, M.S.,
PH.D.**

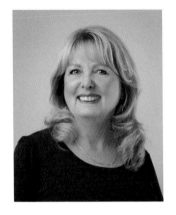

Shelley Metten has been a professor of anatomy at the David Geffen School of Medicine at UCLA for 20 years. Although Dr. Metten enjoys teaching medical school students, she has always had a dream to teach children about their bodies. She believes if kids understand how their bodies are put together and function, they will have the wisdom to make good health choices. Her area of expertise is the reproductive system and so it is particularly important to her that girls and boys have an understanding about how their reproductive system changes during puberty.

Dr. Metten has designed the Anatomy for Kids® series with a dual focus: motivating children and supporting parents. The content of the books is age-appropriate and common threads of knowledge are built from one book to the next. Beginning with a young child's first question about where babies come from until your adolescent has reached sexual maturity, Dr. Metten supports parents through Website resources as well as videos and blogs posted on YouTube and Facebook.

Dr. Metten married her high school sweetheart, Greg, and they have two married children and seven young grandchildren. The questions asked by her adorable grandchildren are a daily reminder of the importance of making her dream a reality for all kids.

**CO-AUTHOR
ALAN ESTRIDGE**

Alan Estridge is a writer, artist, husband, and father. He is also an alumnus of the Animation MFA program at UCLA. The Anatomy for Kids series enables him to bring together a background in biology with a lifelong interest in children's books to relate knowledge in a way that is accessible for all ages.

DESIGN AND ILLUSTRATION

This book is designed under the creative direction of Chris Do, founder of the The Futur and Blind, Inc.

Book Cover, design and anatomical illustrations by Jessie Do. Editorial illustrations by Karen Wang.

ACADEMIC AND PROFESSIONAL CONTRIBUTIONS

CARMINE D. CLEMENTE,
A.B., M.S., PH.D., DR. H.L.
Distinguished Professor of Anatomy and Cell Biology
and Professor of Neurobiology, Emeritus
David Geffen School of Medicine at UCLA
Professor of Surgery (Anatomy)
Charles R. Drew University of Medicine and Science
Los Angeles, California

ALICE CRUZ, M.D.
Internal Medicine
Cedar-Sinai Medical Group
Los Angeles, California

WILLIAM P. MELEGA, PH.D.
Professor, Department of Molecular and Medical
Pharmacology
David Geffen School of Medicine at UCLA
Los Angeles, California

QUYNH PHAM, M.D
Professor, Department of Medicine Division of PMR
David Geffen School of Medicine at UCLA
Los Angeles, California

ANDREA J. RAPKIN, M.D.
Professor, Department of Obstetrics and Gynecology
David Geffen School of Medicine at UCLA
Los Angeles, California

S. ANDREW SCHWARTZ, M.D.
Associate Professor, Department of Orthopaedic Surgery
David Geffen School of Medicine at UCLA
Los Angeles, California

NANCY WAYNE, PH.D.
Professor, Department of Physiology
David Geffen School of Medicine at UCLA
Los Angeles, California

SHAHRAM YAZDANI, M.D.
Professor, Department of Pediatrics
David Geffen School of Medicine at UCLA
Los Angeles, California

Special Thank You

Co-Author	Alan Estridge is a person of inspiration, tremendous creative talent, and a very dear friend.
Junior Editors	Allison Colwell, Emma Cruz, Katherine Pregler, Claire Pregler, Melody Yazdani
Blind	Chris Do is the Founder and Strategic Director of Blind Inc. and The Futur. He has inspired me to think like a storyteller and develop a larger vision for myself as a communicator and author. Also, a special thank you to Jessie Do, the anatomy illustrator and collaborator in the production of this book. Her talent and creative expertise have been the visual foundation of the book.

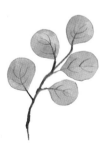